Keto Vegetarian Meals

Nourishment and Health

for your Mind and Body

Lauren Bellisario

Table of Contents

Almond English Muffins

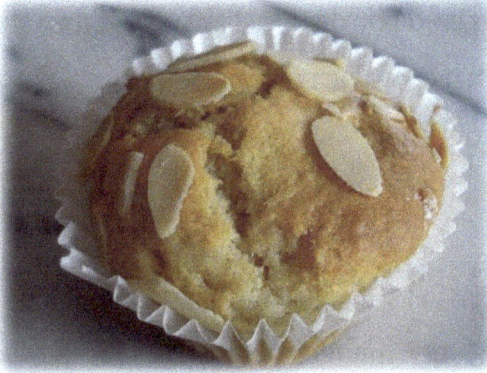

Preparation time: 10 minutes

Cooking time: 10 minutes

Serving: 4

Nutritional Values (Per Serving):

- Calories: 263,
- Total Fat: 26.4g,
- Saturated Fat:9.5 g,
- Total Carbs: 4 g,
- Dietary Fiber: 4g,
- Sugar:3 g,

- Protein:4 g,
- Sodium: 826mg

Ingredients:
- 2 tbsp flax seed powder + 6 tbsp water 2 tbsp almond flour
- ½ tsp baking powder 1 pinch salt
- 3 tbsp butter

Directions:
1. In a small bowl, mix the flax seed with water and allow thickening for 5 minutes.
2. In another bowl, evenly combine the almond flour, baking powder, and salt. Then, pour in the flax egg and whisk again. Let the batter sit for 5 minutes to set.
3. Melt the butter in a frying pan over medium heat and add the mixture in four dollops with 1-inch intervals between each dollop. Fry until golden brown on one side, flip with a spatula and fry further until golden brown.
4. Plate the muffins and serve warm.

Creamy Coconut-Sesame Bread

Preparation time: 10 minutes

Cooking time: 30 minutes

Serving: 4

Nutritional Values (Per Serving):

Calories: 263,

Total Fat: 26.4g,

Saturated Fat: 8.8g,

Total Carbs: 4 g,

Dietary Fiber: 1g,

Sugar: 3g,

Protein:4 g,

Sodium: 826mg

Ingredients:

- 4 tbsp flax seed powder + 1 ½ cups water 2/3 cup cream cheese
- 4 tbsp sesame oil + extra for brushing 1 cup coconut flour
- 2 tbsp psyllium husk powder 1 tsp salt
- 1 tsp baking powder 1 tbsp sesame seeds

Directions:

1. Preheat the oven to 400 F.
2. In a medium bowl, mix the flax seed powder with water and allow soaking for 5 minutes.
3. Whisk in the cream cheese and sesame oil until well mixed.
4. Mix in the coconut flour, psyllium husk powder, salt, and baking powder until adequately combined.
5. Grease a 9 x 5 inches baking tray with cooking spray and spread the dough in the tray. Allow the mixture to stand for 5 minutes and then brush with some sesame oil.
6. Sprinkle the sesame seeds on top and bake the dough for 30 minutes or until golden brown on top and set within.
7. Take out the bread and allow cooling for a few minutes. Slice and serve for breakfast.

Gluten Free Asparagus Quiche

Preparation time: 1 hour 10 minutes

Servings: 6

Nutritional Values (Per Serving):

- Calories 225
- Fat 18 g
- Carbohydrates 5 g
- Sugar 3 g
- Protein 11 g
- Cholesterol 153 mg

Ingredients:

- 5 eggs, beaten
- 1 cup Swiss cheese, shredded
- 1/4 tsp thyme

- 1/4 tsp white pepper
- 1 cup almond milk
- 15 asparagus spears, cut woody ends and cut asparagus in half
- 1/4 tsp salt

Directions:

1. Preheat the oven to 350 F.
2. Spray a quiche dish with cooking spray and set aside.
3. In a bowl, beat together eggs, thyme, white pepper, almond milk, and salt.
4. Arrange asparagus in prepared quiche dish then pour egg mixture over asparagus.
5. Sprinkle shredded cheese all over asparagus and egg mixture.
6. Place in preheated oven and bake for 60 minutes.
7. Cut quiche into slices and serve.

Mini Vegetable Quiche

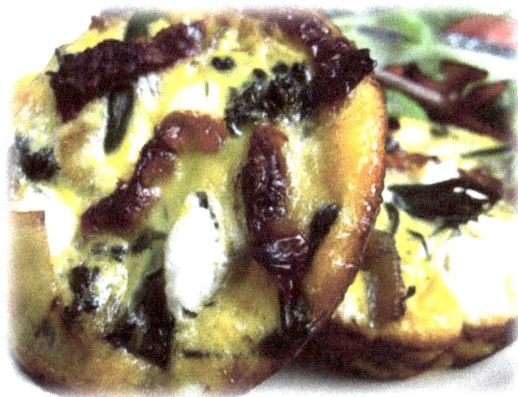

Preparation time: 30 minutes

Servings: 12

Nutritional Values (per Serving):

- Calories 73
- Fat 5 g
- Carbohydrates 1 g
- Sugar 0.6 g
- Protein 5 g
- Cholesterol 103 mg

Ingredients:

- 7 eggs
- 1/4 cup onion, chopped
- 1/4 cup mushroom, diced
- 1/4 cup bell pepper, diced
- 3/4 cup cheddar cheese, shredded
- 10 oz frozen spinach, chopped

Directions:

1. Line muffin cups with aluminum foil cups set aside.
2. Add all ingredients into the large bowl and beat lightly to combine.
3. Pour egg mixture into the prepared muffin tray.
4. Bake at 350 F for 20 minutes.
5. Serve warm and enjoy.

Simple Roasted Radishes

Preparation time: 45 minutes

Servings: 2

Nutritional Valuee (per Serving):

- Calories 220
- Fat 21 g
- Carbohydrates 8 g
- Sugar 3 g
- Protein 1 g
- Cholesterol 0 mg

Ingredients:

- 3 cups radish, clean and halved
- 3 tbsp olive oil
- 2 tbsp fresh rosemary, chopped
- 10 black peppercorns, crushed
- 2 tsp sea salt

Directions:

1. Preheat the oven to 425 F.
2. Add radishes, salt, peppercorns, rosemary, and 2 tablespoons of olive oil in a bowl and toss well.
3. Pour radishes mixture into the baking sheet and bake in preheated oven for 30 minutes.
4. Heat remaining olive oil in a pan over medium heat.
5. Add baked radishes in the pan and sauté for 2 minutes.
6. Serve immediately and enjoy.

Coconut Broccoli Cheese Loaf

Preparation time: 35 minutes

Servings: 5

Nutritional Values (per Serving):

Calories 209

Fat 13 g

Carbohydrates 8 g

Sugar 1 g

Protein 13 g

Cholesterol 187 mg

Ingredients:

- 5 eggs, lightly beaten
- 2 tsp baking powder
- 3 1/1 tbsp coconut flour

- 3/4 cup broccoli florets, chopped
- 1 cup cheddar cheese, shredded
- 1 tsp salt

Directions:

1. Preheat the oven to 350 F.
2. Spray a loaf pan with cooking spray and set aside.
3. Add all ingredients into the bowl and mix well.
4. Pour egg mixture into the prepared loaf pan and bake in preheated oven for 30 minutes.
5. Cut loaf into the slices and serve.

Green Parsley Broccoli Cauliflower Puree

Preparation time: 35 minutes

Servings: 4

Nutritional Values (per Serving):

- Calories 154
- Fat 12 g
- Carbohydrates 7 g
- Sugar 2 g
- Protein 5 g
- Cholesterol 31 mg

Ingredients:

- 1 1/3 small broccoli, cut into florets
- 4 tbsp fresh parsley
- 1 small cauliflower, cut into florets
- 2 cups vegetable broth

- 4 tbsp butter
- 1 tsp sea salt

Directions:

1. Add cauliflower and broccoli in steamer and steam for 15 minutes.
2. Add steamed cauliflower and broccoli in a blender with butter, broth, and parsley and blend until smooth.
3. Season puree with salt and serve.

Healthy Braised Garlic Kale

Preparation time: 50 minutes

Servings: 4

Nutritional Values (per Serving):

- Calories 172
- Fat 14 g
- Carbohydrates 11 g
- Sugar 1 g
- Protein 2 g
- Cholesterol 0 mg

Ingredients:

- 10 oz kale, stems removed and chopped
- 2 cups vegetable stock
- 4 tbsp coconut oil
- 1 tsp chili pepper flakes, dried
- 1 medium onion, sliced

- 4 garlic cloves, minced
- 1 tsp sea salt

Directions:

1. Heat coconut oil in a pan over medium heat.
2. Once the oil is hot then add onion, garlic and chili pepper flakes and sauté until lightly brown.
3. Pour vegetable stock and stir well.
4. Now add chopped kale and season with salt. Stir well.
5. Cover pan with lid and cook on low heat for 40 minutes.
6. Serve and enjoy.

Lime Basil Cucumbers

Preparation time: 15 minutes

Servings: 4

Nutritional Values (per Serving):

- Calories 85
- Fat 7 g
- Carbohydrates 6 g
- Sugar 2 g
- Protein 1 g
- Cholesterol 0 mg

Ingredients:

- 2 medium cucumber, remove seeds and diced
- 1 tsp basil leaves, chopped
- 1 tsp fresh lime juice
- 2 tsp turmeric powder

- 2 tbsp coconut oil
- 1/4 tsp sea salt

Directions:

1. Heat coconut oil in a pan over medium heat.
2. Once the oil is hot then, add turmeric powder and basil leaves and stir for 1 minute.
3. Now add cucumber, lime juice, and salt. Stir well.
4. Serve and enjoy.

Yummy Cheese Grits

Preparation time: 10 minutes

Servings: 4

Nutritional Values (per Serving):

- Calories 408
- Fat 37 g
- Carbohydrates 1 g
- Sugar 1 g
- Protein 17 g
- Cholesterol 448 mg

Ingredients:

- 8 large eggs
- 1/2 cup cheddar cheese, shredded
- 1/2 cup butter
- 1/2 cup vegetable broth
- 1 tsp sea salt

Directions:

1. In a bowl, whisk together eggs, salt, and broth.
2. Melt butter in a saucepan over medium heat.
3. Add egg mixture to the saucepan and cook until thickens.
4. Once the mixture is thickened and curds formed then add shredded cheese and stir well to combine.
5. Serve warm and enjoy.

Creamy Egg Salad

Preparation time: 15 minutes

Servings: 4

Nutritional Values (per Serving):

- Calories 367
- Fat 28 g
- Carbohydrates 12 g
- Sugar 4 g
- Protein 17 g
- Cholesterol 503 mg

Ingredients:

- 12 eggs, hard-boiled
- 1 scallion, sliced
- 1/2 cup celery, diced
- 1 tbsp Dijon mustard

- 3/4 cup mayonnaise Pepper
- Salt

Directions:

1. Separate egg yolks and egg whites.
2. Chop egg whites into the small pieces.
3. Add egg yolks, salt, mustard, and mayonnaise in a blender and blend until smooth.
4. Add chopped egg whites, scallion and celery in a large bowl then add egg yolk mixture and mix well.
5. Season with pepper and salt.
6. Serve and enjoy.

Peppers Rice

Preparation time: 10 minutes

Cooking time: 25 minutes

Servings: 4

Nutritional Values (Per Serving):

- Calories 69
- Fat 4.4
- Fiber 1.3
- Carbs 8.9
- Protein 1.3

Ingredients:

- 1 yellow bell pepper, chopped
- 1 red bell pepper, chopped
- 1 green bell pepper, chopped

- 4 scallions, chopped
- 2 cups cauliflower rice 1 cup vegetable stock
- 1 tablespoon olive oil
- 1 teaspoon coriander, ground
- 1 teaspoon cumin, ground
- 1 teaspoon basil, dried
- 1 teaspoon oregano, dried
- A pinch of salt and black pepper
- 1 tablespoon chives, chopped

Directions:

1. Heat up a pan with the oil over medium heat, add the scallions and the peppers and sauté for 5 minutes.
2. Add the cauliflower rice and the other ingredients, toss, cook over medium heat for 20 minutes, divide between plates and serve as a side dish.

Cauliflower and Chives Mash

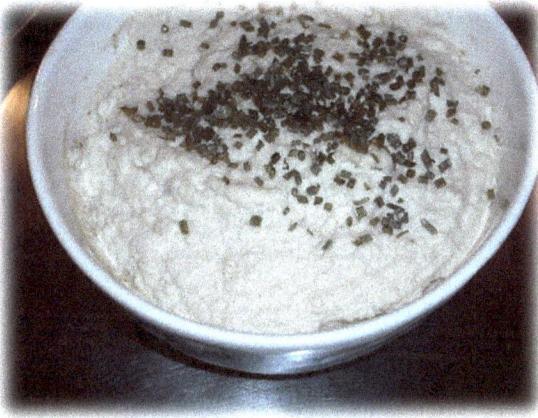

Preparation time: 10 minutes

Cooking time: 20 minutes

Servings: 4

Nutritional Values (Per Serving):

- Calories 200
- Fat 14.7
- Fiber 7.2
- Carbs 16.3
- Protein 6.1

Ingredients:

- 2 pounds cauliflower florets
- 2 cups water
- 1 teaspoon thyme, dried
- 1 teaspoon cumin, dried
- 1 cup coconut cream
- 2 garlic cloves, minced
- A pinch of salt and black pepper

Directions:

1. Put the cauliflower florets in a pot, add the water and the other ingredients except the cream, bring to a simmer and cook over medium heat for 20 minutes.
2. Drain the cauliflower, add the cream, mash everything with a potato masher, whisk well, divide between plates and serve.

Baked Artichokes and Green Beans

Preparation time: 10 minutes

Cooking time: 40 minutes

Servings: 4

Nutritional Values (Per Serving):

- Calories 132
- Fat 7.8
- Fiber 6.9
- Carbs 14.8
- Protein 4.4

Ingredients:

- 1 pound green beans, trimmed and halved
- 3 scallions, chopped
- 2 tablespoons olive oil

- 1 cup canned artichoke hearts, drained and quartered
- 2 garlic cloves, minced
- 1/3 cup tomato passata
- A pinch of salt and black pepper
- 2 teaspoons mustard powder
- 1 teaspoon cumin, ground
- 1 teaspoon coriander, ground

Directions:

1. Heat up a pan with the oil over medium heat, add the scallions and the garlic and sauté for 5 minutes.
2. Add the green beans and the other ingredients, toss, introduce in the oven and bake at 390 degrees F for 35 minutes.
3. Divide the mix between plates and serve as a side dish.

Cumin Cauliflower Rice and Broccoli

Preparation time: 10 minutes

Cooking time: 25 minutes

Servings: 4

Nutritional Values (Per Serving):

- Calories 81
- Fat 7.9
- Fiber 1.5
- Carbs 4.1
- Protein 1.1

Ingredients:

- 2 cups cauliflower rice
- 1 cup broccoli florets
- 2 tablespoons olive oil

- 4 scallions, chopped
- 1 teaspoon sweet paprika
- 1 teaspoon chili powder
- 1 cup vegetable stock
- 1 teaspoon red pepper flakes
- A pinch of salt and black pepper
- ¼ teaspoon cumin, ground

Directions:

1. Heat up a pan with the oil over medium heat, add the scallions, paprika and chili powder and sauté for 5 minutes.
2. Add the cauliflower rice and the other ingredients, toss, bring to a simmer, cook over medium heat for 20 minutes, divide between plates and serve.

Turmeric Cauliflower Rice and Tomatoes

Preparation time: 10 minutes

Cooking time: 25 minutes

Servings: 4

Nutritional Values (Per Serving):

- Calories 77
- Fat 7.7
- Fiber 1
- Carbs 3.7
- Protein 0.7

Ingredients:

- 2 tablespoons olive oil
- 2 cups cauliflower rice
- 2 scallions, chopped

- 2 garlic cloves, minced
- 1 cup cherry tomatoes, halved
- 1 teaspoon basil, dried
- 1 teaspoon oregano, dried
- A pinch of salt and black pepper
- ¼ teaspoon turmeric powder
- 1 cup vegetable stock
- A handful cilantro, chopped

Directions:

1. Heat up a pan with the oil over medium heat, add the scallions, garlic, basil, oregano and turmeric and sauté for 5 minutes.
2. Add the cauliflower rice, tomatoes and the remaining ingredients, toss, cook over medium heat for 20 minutes, divide between plates and serve as a side dish.

Flavored Tomato and Okra Mix

Preparation time: 10 minutes

Cooking time: 30 minutes

Servings: 6

Nutritional Values (Per Serving):

- Calories 84
- Fat 2.1
- Fiber 5.4
- Carbs 14.8
- Protein 4

Ingredients:

- 1 cup scallions, chopped
- 1 pound cherry tomatoes, halved
- 2 cups okra, sliced
- 2 tablespoons avocado oil
- 4 garlic cloves, chopped

- 2 teaspoons oregano, dried
- A pinch of salt and black pepper
- 2 teaspoons cumin, ground
- 1 cup veggie stock
- 2 tablespoons tomato passata

Directions:

1. Heat up a pan with the oil over medium heat, add the scallions and the garlic and sauté for 5 minutes.
2. Add the tomatoes, the okra and the other ingredients, toss, cook over medium heat for 25 minutes, divide between plates and serve as a side dish.

Orange Scallions and Brussels Sprouts

Preparation time: 10 minutes

Cooking time: 25 minutes

Servings: 4

Nutritional Values (Per Serving):

- Calories 193
- Fat 4
- Fiber 1
- Carbs 8
- Protein 10

Ingredients:

- 1 pound Brussels sprouts, trimmed and halved
- 1 cup scallions, chopped
- Zest of 1 lime, grated

- 1 tablespoon olive oil
- ¼ cup orange juice
- 2 tablespoons stevia
- A pinch of salt and black pepper

Directions:

1. Heat up a pan with the oil over medium heat, add the scallions and sauté for 5 minutes.
2. Add the sprouts and the other ingredients, toss, cook over medium heat for 20 minutes more, divide the mix between plates and serve.

Spinach Soup

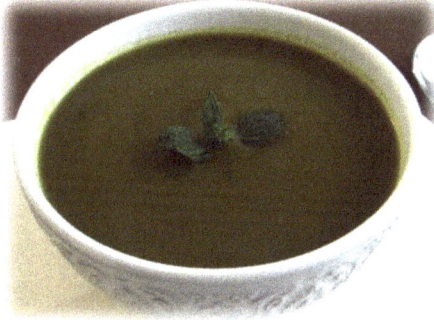

Preparation time: 10 minutes

Cooking time: 15 minutes

Servings: 8

Nutritional Values (Per Serving):

- Calories – 245
- Fat – 24
- Fiber – 3
- Carbs – 4
- Protein - 6

Ingredients:

- 2 tablespoons butter
- 20 ounces spinach, chopped
- 1 teaspoon garlic, minced
- Salt and ground black pepper, to taste
- 45 ounces chicken stock
- ½ teaspoon ground nutmeg
- 2 cups heavy cream
- 1 onion, peeled and chopped

Directions:

1. Heat up a pot with the butter over medium heat, add the onion, stir, and cook for 4 minutes.
2. Add the garlic, stir, and cook for 1 minute.
3. Add the spinach and stock, stir, and cook for 5 minutes.
4. Blend soup with an immersion blender, and heat up the soup again.
5. Add the salt, pepper, nutmeg, and cream, stir, and cook for 5 minutes.
6. Ladle into bowls and serve.

Sautéed Mustard Greens

Preparation time: 5 minutes

Cooking time: 15 minutes

Servings: 4

Nutritional Values (Per Serving):

- Calories – 120
- Fat – 3
- Fiber – 1
- Carbs – 3
- Protein - 6

Ingredients:

- 2 garlic cloves, peeled and minced
- 1 pound mustard greens, torn
- 1 tablespoon olive oil
- ½ cup onion, sliced
- Salt and ground black pepper, to taste

- 3 tablespoons vegetable stock
- ¼ teaspoon dark sesame oil

Directions:

1. Heat up a pan with the oil over medium heat, add the onions, stir, and brown them for 10 minutes.
2. Add the garlic, stir, and cook for 1 minute.
3. Add the stock, greens, salt, and pepper, stir, and cook for 5 minutes.
4. Add more salt and pepper, and sesame oil, toss to coat, divide on plates, and serve.

Collard Greens and Poached Eggs

Preparation time: 10 minutes

Cooking time: 15 minutes

Servings: 6

Nutritional Values (Per Serving):

- Calories – 245
- Fat – 20
- Fiber – 1
- Carbs – 5
- Protein - 12

Ingredients:

- 1 tablespoon chipotle in adobo, mashed
- 6 eggs
- 3 tablespoons butter
- 1 onion, peeled and chopped
- 2 garlic cloves, peeled and minced

- 6 bacon slices, chopped
- 3 bunches collard greens, chopped
- ½ cup chicken stock
- Salt and ground black pepper, to taste
- 1 tablespoon lime juice
- Cheddar cheese, grated, for serving

Directions:

1. Heat up a pan over medium-high heat, add the bacon, cook until crispy, transfer to paper towels, drain grease, and leave aside.
2. Heat up the pan again over medium heat, add the garlic and onion, stir, and cook for 2 minutes.
3. Return the bacon to the pan, stir, and cook for 3 minutes.
4. Add the chipotle in adobo paste, collard greens, salt, and pepper, stir, and cook for 10 minutes.
5. Add the stock and lime juice, and stir.
6. Make 6 holes in collard greens mixture, divide butter in them, crack an egg in each hole, cover the pan, and cook until eggs are done.
7. Divide this on plates and serve with cheddar cheese sprinkled on top.

Collard Greens Soup

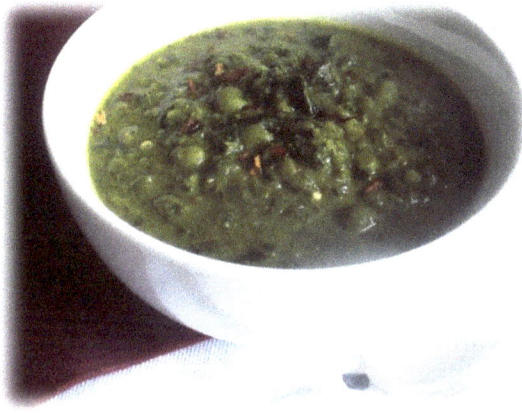

Preparation time: 10 minutes

Cooking time: 40 minutes

Servings: 12

Nutritional Values (Per Serving):

- Calories – 150
- Fat – 3
- Fiber – 2
- Carbs – 4
- Protein – 8

Ingredients:

- 1 teaspoon chili powder
- 1 tablespoon avocado oil
- 2 teaspoons smoked paprika
- 1 teaspoon cumin
- 1 onion, peeled and chopped
- A pinch of red pepper flakes
- 10 cups water
- 3 celery stalks, chopped
- 3 carrots, peeled and chopped
- 15 ounces canned diced tomatoes
- 2 tablespoons tamari sauce
- 6 ounces canned tomato paste
- 2 tablespoons lemon juice
- Salt and ground black pepper, to taste
- 6 cups collard greens, stems discarded
- 1 tablespoon swerve
- 1 teaspoon dried garlic
- 1 tablespoon herb seasoning

Directions:

1. Heat up a pot with the oil over medium-high heat, add the cumin, pepper flakes, paprika, and chili powder, and stir well.
2. Add the celery, onion, and carrots, stir, and cook for 10 minutes.
3. Add the tamari sauce, tomatoes, tomato paste, water, lemon juice, salt, pepper, herb seasoning, swerve, garlic granules, and collard greens, stir, bring to a boil, cover, and cook for 30 minutes.
4. Stir again, ladle into bowls, and serve.

Spring Greens Soup

Preparation time: 10 minutes

Cooking time: 30 minutes

Servings: 4

Nutritional Values (Per Serving):

- Calories – 140
- Fat – 2
- Fiber – 1
- Carbs – 3
- Protein - 7

Ingredients:

- 2 cups mustard greens, chopped
- 2 cups collard greens, chopped
- 3 quarts vegetable stock
- 1 onion, peeled and chopped
- Salt and ground black pepper, to taste

- 2 tablespoons coconut aminos
- 2 teaspoons fresh ginger, grated

Directions:

1. Put the stock into a pot, and bring to a simmer over medium-high heat.
2. Add the mustard, collard greens, onion, salt, pepper, coconut aminos, and ginger, stir, cover the pot, and cook for 30 minutes.
3. Blend the soup using an immersion blender, add more salt, and pepper, heat up over medium heat, ladle into soup bowls, and serve.

Quick Thai Coconut Mushroom Soup

Preparation time: 5 Minutes

Cooking time: 10 Minutes

Servings: 4

Ingredients:

- 1½ cups low-sodium vegetable broth, divided
- 2 garlic cloves, minced
- 1 tablespoon minced fresh ginger
- 1 (8-ounce) package baby bella or white button mushrooms, stemmed and sliced
- 1 (13.5-ounce) can full-fat coconut milk
- Juice of ½ lemon
- Juice of ½ lime
- 2 tablespoons chopped fresh Thai basil
- 1 tablespoon chopped fresh cilantro

- Fresh cilantro leaves, for garnish (optional)
- Lime wedges, for garnish (optional)

Directions:

1. Preparing the ingredients.
2. Heat ½ cup of broth in a large saucepot over medium-high heat. Sauté the garlic and ginger in the broth for 1 minute, or until fragrant.
3. Add the mushrooms and slowly pour in the remaining 1 cup of broth. Bring to a boil and reduce the heat to a simmer. Add the coconut milk, lemon juice, lime juice, basil, and chopped cilantro.
4. Let simmer for 5 minutes, or until heated through. Garnish with whole cilantro leaves and lime wedges, if desired.

Chilled Avocado-Tomato Soup

Preparation time: 15 Minutes

Cooking time: 0 Minutes

Servings: 4

Ingredients:

- 2 garlic cloves, crushed
- Salt
- 2 ripe Hass avocados
- 2 teaspoons lemon juice
- 2 pounds ripe plum tomatoes, coarsely chopped
- 1 (14.5-ounce) can crushed tomatoes
- 1 cup tomato juice
- Freshly ground black pepper
- 8 fresh basil leaves, for garnish

Directions:

1. In a blender or food processor, combine the garlic and 1⁄2 teaspoon of salt and process to a paste. Pit and peel one of the avocados and add it to the food processor along with the lemon juice. Process until smooth. Add the fresh and canned tomatoes, tomato juice, and salt and pepper to taste. Process until smooth.

2. Transfer the soup to a large container, cover, and refrigerate until chilled, 2 to 3 hours.

3. Taste, adjusting seasonings if necessary. Pit and peel the remaining avocado and cut it into a small dice. Slice the basil leaves into thin strips. Ladle the soup into bowls, add the diced avocado, garnish with basil, and serve.

Spicy Black Bean Orzo Soup

Preparation time: 5 Minutes

Cooking time: 50 Minutes

Servings: 4 To 6

Ingredients:

- 2 tablespoons olive oil
- 3 garlic cloves, minced
- 1 tablespoon chili powder
- 1 teaspoon dried oregano
- 4½ cups cooked or 3 (15.5-ounce) cans black beans, drained and rinsed
- 1 small jalapeño, seeded and finely chopped (optional)
- ¼ cup minced oil-packed sun-dried tomatoes
- 4 cups vegetable broth (homemade, -bought, or water)
- 1 cup water
- Salt and freshly ground black peppe

- ½ cup orzo
- 2 tablespoons chopped fresh cilantro, for garnish

Directions:

1. In a large soup pot, heat the oil over medium heat. Add the garlic and cook until fragrant, about 1 minute. Stir in the chili powder, oregano, beans, jalapeño, if using, tomatoes, broth, water, and salt and pepper to taste. Simmer for 30 minutes to blend flavors.

2. Puree the soup in the pot with an immersion blender or in a blender or food processor, in batches if necessary, and return to the pot. Cook the soup 15 minutes longer over medium heat. Taste, adjusting seasonings, and add more water if necessary.

3. While the soup is simmering, cook the orzo in a pot of boiling salted water, stirring occasionally, until al dente, about 5 minutes. Drain the orzo and divide it among the soup bowls. Ladle the soup into the bowls, garnish with cilantro, and serve.

Pesto Parmesan Tempeh with Green Pasta

Preparation time: 1 hour 27 minutes

Serving: 4

Nutritional Values (Per Serving):

- Calories:442
- Total Fat:29.4g
- Saturated Fat:11.3g
- Total Carbs:8g
- Dietary Fiber:1g
- Sugar:1g
- Protein:39g
- Sodium:814mg

Ingredients:

- 4 tempeh
- Salt and black pepper to taste
- ½ cup basil pesto, olive oil-based
- 1 cup grated parmesan cheese
- 1 tbsp butter
- 4 large turnips, Blade C, noodle trimmed

Directions:

1. Preheat the oven to 350 F.
2. Season the tempeh with salt, black pepper and place on a baking sheet. Divide the pesto on top and spread well on the tempeh.
3. Place the sheet in the oven and bake for 45 minutes to 1 hour or until cooked through.
4. When ready, pull out the baking sheet and divide half of the parmesan cheese on top of the tempeh. Cook further for 10 minutes or until the cheese melts. Remove the tempeh and set aside for serving.
5. Melt the butter in a medium skillet and sauté the turnips until tender, 5 to 7 minutes. Stir in the remaining parmesan cheese and divide between serving plates.
6. Top with the tempeh and serve warm.

Ruby Grapefruit and Radicchio Salad

Preparation time: 10 Minutes

Cooking time: 0 Minutes

Servings: 4

Ingredients:

For the Salad

- 1 large ruby grapefruit
- 1 small head radicchio, torn into bite-size pieces
- 2 cups green leaf lettuce, torn into bite-size pieces
- 2 cups baby spinach
- 1 bunch watercress
- 4 to 6 radishes, sliced paper-thin

For The Dressing

- juice of 1 lemon
- 2 teaspoons agave
- 1 teaspoon white wine vinegar
- ½ teaspoon sea salt
- ½ teaspoon freshly ground black pepper
- ¼ cup extra-virgin olive oil

Directions:

1. To make the salad: Cut both ends off of the grapefruit, stand it on a cutting board on one of the flat sides, and, using a sharp knife, cut away the peel and all of the white pith. Remove the individual segments by slicing between the membrane and fruit on each side of each segment, dropping the fruit into a large salad bowl as you go. Add the radicchio, lettuce, spinach, watercress, and radishes to the bowl and toss well.

2. To make the dressing: Whisk together the lemon juice, agave, vinegar, salt, and pepper. Slowly whisk in the olive oil until the mixture is well combined and emulsified. Toss the salad with the dressing and serve immediately.

Darn Good Caesar Salad

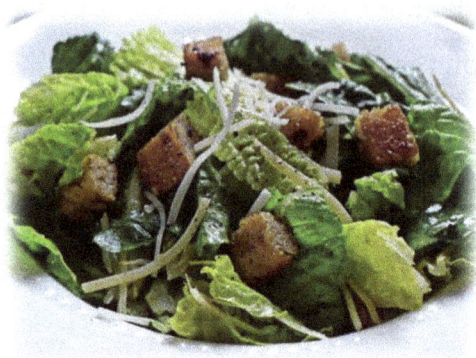

Preparation time: 10 Minutes

Cooking time: 0 Minutes

Servings: 4

Ingredients:

For the Dressing

- ½ cup walnuts
- ½ cup water
- 3 tablespoons olive oil
- Juice of ½ lime
- 1 tablespoon white miso paste

- 1 teaspoon soy sauce or gluten-free tamari
- 1 teaspoon Dijon mustard
- 1 teaspoon garlic powder
- ¼ teaspoon sea salt
- ½ teaspoon black pepper

For the Salad

- 2 heads romaine lettuce, chopped
- 1 cup cherry tomatoes, halved
- Walnut Parmesan or store-bought vegan Parmesan, for garnish
- Vegan croutons, for garnish (optional)

Directions:

1. To make the dressing: In a blender, combine all the dressing ingredients and blend until almost smooth, about 2 minutes. It's okay if this dressing is slightly chunky, which is more like a classic Caesar dressing texture.
2. To make the salad: In a large bowl, toss the lettuce with half of the dressing. Add more as desired. Divide among serving plates and top with the tomatoes and Parmesan. Finish the salad off with croutons, if desired.

Potato Salad Redux

Preparation time: 5 Minutes

Cooking time: 30 Minutes

Servings: 4 To 6

Ingredients:

- 1½ pounds small white potatoes, unpeeled
- 2 celery ribs, cut into ¼-inch slices
- ¼ cup sweet pickle relish
- 3 tablespoons minced green onions
- ½ to ¾ cup vegan mayonnaise, homemade or store-bought
- 1 tablespoon soy milk
- 1 tablespoon tarragon vinegar
- 1 teaspoon Dijon mustard
- ½ teaspoon salt (optional)
- Freshly ground black pepper

Directions:

1. In a large pot of salted boiling water, cook the potatoes until just tender, about 30 minutes. Drain and set aside to cool. When cool enough to handle, peel the potatoes and cut them into 1-inch dice. Transfer the potatoes to a large bowl and add the celery, pickle relish, and green onions. Set aside.

2. In a small bowl, combine the mayonnaise, soy milk, vinegar, mustard, salt, and pepper to taste. Mix until well blended. Pour the dressing onto the potato mixture, toss gently to combine, and serve.

Apple and Ginger Slaw

Preparation time: 10 Minutes

Cooking time: 0 Minutes

Servings: 4

Ingredients:

- 2 tablespoons olive oil
- juice of 1 lemon, or 2 tablespoons prepared lemon juice
- 1 teaspoon grated fresh ginger
- pinch of sea salt
- 2 apples, peeled and julienned
- 4 cups shredded red cabbage

Directions:

1. In a small bowl, whisk together the olive oil, lemon juice, ginger, and salt and set aside.
2. In a large bowl, combine the apples and cabbage.

3. Toss with the vinaigrette and serve immediately. Store leftovers in an airtight container in the refrigerator for up to 3 days.

Loaded Baked Potatoes

Preparation time: 10 minutes

Cooking time: 32 minutes

Servings: 2

Nutritional Values (Per Serving):

- Calories: 422 Cal
- Fat: 16 g
- Carbs: 59 g
- Protein: 9 g
- Fiber: 6 g

Ingredients:

- 1/2 cup cooked chickpeas
- 2 medium potatoes, scrubbed
- 1 cup broccoli florets, steamed

- 1/4 cup vegan bacon bits
- 2 tablespoons all-purpose seasoning
- ¼ cup vegan cheese sauce
- 1/2 cup vegan sour cream

Directions:

1. Pierce hole in the potatoes, microwave them for 12 minutes over high heat setting until soft to touch, and then bake them for 20 minutes at 450 degrees f until very tender.
2. Open the potatoes, mash the flesh with a fork, then top evenly with remaining ingredients and serve.

Coconut Rice

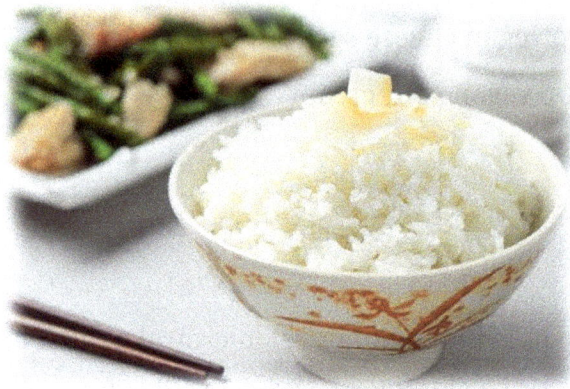

Preparation time: 5 minutes

Cooking time: 20 minutes

Servings: 4

Nutritional Values (Per Serving):

- Calories:453 Cal
- Fat: 21 g
- Carbs: 61.4 g
- Protein: 6.8 g
- Fiber: 2 g

Ingredients:

- 1 1/2 cups white rice
- 1 teaspoon coconut sugar
- 1/8 teaspoon salt
- 14 ounces coconut milk, unsweetened
- 1 1/4 cups water

Directions:

1. Take a saucepan, place it over medium heat, add all the ingredients in it, stir well and bring the mixture to a boil.
2. Switch heat to medium-low level, simmer the rice for 20 minutes until tender, and then serve straight away.

Zucchini and Amaranth Patties

Preparation time: 10 minutes

Cooking time: 30 minutes

Servings: 14

Nutritional Values (Per Serving):

- Calories:152 Cal
- Fat: 3 g
- Carbs: 29 g
- Protein: 7 g
- Fiber: 6 g

Ingredients:

- 1 1/2 cups shredded zucchini
- ½ of a medium onion, shredded
- 1 1/2 cups cooked white beans
- 1/2 cup amaranth seeds
- 1 teaspoon red chili powder

- 1/2 teaspoon cumin
- 1/2 cup cornmeal
- 1/4 cup flax meal
- 1 tablespoon salsa
- 1 1/2 cups vegetable broth

Directions:

1. Stir together stock and amaranth on a pot, bring it to a boil over medium-high heat, then switch heat to medium-low level and simmer until all the liquid is absorbed.
2. Mash the white beans in a bowl, add remaining ingredients including cooked amaranth and stir until well mixed.
3. Shape the mixture into patties, then place them on a baking sheet lined with parchment sheet and bake for 30 minutes until browned and crispy, turning halfway.
4. Serve straight away.

Rice Pizza

Preparation time: 10 minutes

Cooking time: 35 minutes

Servings: 6

Nutritional Values (Per Serving):

- Calories: 1 Cal
- Fat: 5 g
- Carbs: 30 g
- Protein: 3 g
- Fiber: 1 g

Ingredients:

For the crust:

- 1 1/2 cup short-grain rice, cooked
- 1/2 teaspoon garlic powder
- 1 teaspoon coconut sugar
- 1 tablespoon red chili flakes

For the sauce:

- 1/4 teaspoon onion powder
- 1 tablespoon nutritional yeast
- 1/4 teaspoon garlic powder
- 1/4 teaspoon ginger powder
- 1 tablespoon red chili flakes
- 1 teaspoon soy sauce
- 1/2 cup tomato purée

For the toppings:

- 2 1/2 cups oyster mushrooms
- 1 chili pepper, deseeded, sliced
- 2 scallions, sliced
- 1 teaspoon coconut sugar
- 1 teaspoon soy sauce
- Baby corn as needed

Directions:

1. Prepare the crust and for this, place all of its ingredients in a bowl and stir until well combined.

2. Then take a pizza pan, line it with parchment sheet, place rice mixture in it, spread it evenly, and then bake for 20 minutes at 350 degrees f.

3. Then spread tomato sauce over the crust, top evenly with remaining ingredients for the topping and continue baking for 15 minutes.

4. When done, slice the pizza into wedges and serve.

Quinoa and Black Bean Burgers

Preparation time: 10 minutes

Cooking time: 6 minutes

Servings: 5

Nutritional Values (Per Serving):

- Calories: 245 Cal
- Fat: 10.6 g
- Carbs: 29 g
- Protein: 9.3 g
- Fiber: 7.2 g

Ingredients:

- 1/4 cup quinoa, cooked
- 15 ounces cooked black beans
- 2 tablespoons minced white onion
- 1/4 cup minced bell pepper
- ½ teaspoon minced garlic

- 1/2 teaspoon salt
- 1 1/2 teaspoons ground cumin
- 1/2 cup breadcrumbs
- 1 teaspoon hot pepper sauce
- 3 tablespoons olive oil
- 1 flax egg

Directions:

1. Place all the ingredients in a bowl, except for oil, stir until well combined, and then shape the mixture into five patties.
2. Heat oil in a frying pan over medium heat, add patties and cook for 3 minutes per side until browned.
3. Serve straight away.

Jalapeno and Cilantro Hummus

Preparation time: 5 minutes

Cooking time: 0 minute

Servings: 4

Nutritional Values (Per Serving):

- Calories: 137 Cal
- Fat: 2.3 g
- Carbs: 23.3 g
- Protein: 7.3 g
- Fiber: 6.6 g

Ingredients:

- ½ cup cilantro
- 1 1/2 cups chickpeas, cooked
- 1/2 of jalapeno pepper, sliced
- ½ teaspoon salt
- ½ teaspoon minced garlic

- 1 tablespoon lime juice
- 1/4 cup tahini
- ¼ water

Directions:

1. Place all the ingredients in a bowl and pulse for 2 minutes until smooth.
2. Tip the hummus in a bowl, drizzle with oil sprinkle with cilantro, and then serve.

Berry Cake

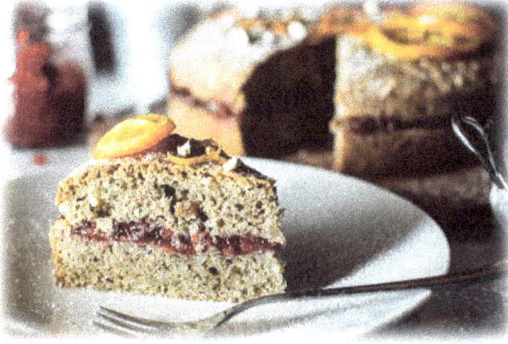

Preparation time: 10 minutes

Cooking time: 30 minutes

Servings: 6

Nutritional Values (Per Serving):

- Calories 225
- Fat 9
- Fiber 4.5

- Carbs 10.2
- Protein 4.5

Ingredients:

- 2 cups coconut flour
- 1 cup blueberries
- 1 cup strawberries, chopped
- 2 tablespoons almonds, chopped
- 2 tablespoons walnuts, chopped
- 3 tablespoons stevia
- 1 teaspoon almond extract
- 3 tablespoons flaxseed mixed with 4 tablespoons water
- ½ cup coconut cream
- 2 tablespoons avocado oil
- 1 teaspoon baking powder
- Cooking spray

Directions:

1. In a bowl, combine the coconut flour with the berries, the nuts, stevia and the other ingredients, and whisk well.

2. Grease a cake pan with the cooking spray, pour the cake mix inside, introduce everything in the oven at 360 degrees F and bake for 30 minutes.
3. Cool the cake down, slice and serve.

Dates Mousse

Preparation time: 30 minutes

Cooking time: 0 minutes

Servings: 4

Nutritional Values (Per Serving):

- Calories 141
- Fat 4.7
- Fiber 4.7
- Carbs 8.3
- Protein 0.8

Ingredients:

- 2 cups coconut cream
- ¼ cup stevia
- 2 cups dates, chopped
- 1 teaspoon almond extract
- 1 teaspoon vanilla extract

Directions:

1. In a blender, combine the cream with the stevia, dates and the other ingredients, pulse well, divide into cups and keep in the fridge for 30 minutes before serving.

Minty Almond Cups

Preparation time: 10 minutes

Cooking time: 10 minutes

Servings: 4

Nutritional Values (Per Serving):

- Calories 135
- Fat 4.1
- Fiber 3.8
- Carbs 4.1
- Protein 2.3

Ingredients:

- 1 cup almonds, roughly chopped
- 1 tablespoon mint, chopped
- ½ cup coconut cream
- 2 tablespoons stevia
- 1 teaspoon vanilla extract

Directions:

1. In a pan, combine the almonds with the mint, the cream and the other ingredients, whisk, simmer over medium heat for 10 minutes, divide into cups and serve cold.

Lime Cake

Preparation time: 10 minutes

Cooking time: 40 minutes

Servings: 4

Nutritional Values (Per Serving):

- Calories 186
- Fat 16.4
- Fiber 3
- Carbs 6.8
- Protein 4.7

Ingredients:

- ½ cup almonds, chopped
- Zest of 1 lime grated
- Juice of 1 lime
- 1 cup stevia
- 2 tablespoons flaxseed mixed with 3 tablespoons water

- 1 teaspoon vanilla extract
- 1 and ½ cup almond flour
- ½ cup coconut cream
- 1 teaspoon baking soda

Directions:

In a bowl, combine the almond with the lime zest, lime juice and the other ingredients, whisk well and pour into a cake pan lined with parchment paper.

Introduce in the oven at 360 degrees F, bake for 40 minutes, cool down, slice and serve.

Vanilla Pudding

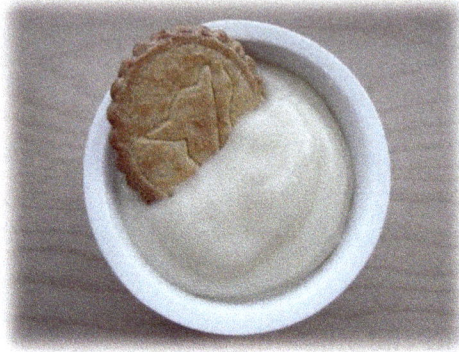

Preparation time: 10 minutes

Cooking time: 40 minutes

Servings: 4

Nutritional Values (Per Serving):

- Calories 399
- Fat 39.3
- Fiber 4.7
- Carbs 11.2
- Protein 7.2

Ingredients:

- 2 cups almond flour
- 3 tablespoons walnuts, chopped
- 1 and ½ cups coconut cream
- 3 tablespoons flaxseed mixed with 4 tablespoons water
- 1 cup stevia
- 1 teaspoon vanilla extract
- 1 teaspoon baking powder
- 1 teaspoon nutmeg, ground

Directions:

1. In a bowl, combine the flour with the walnuts, the cream and the other ingredients, whisk well and pour into 4 ramekins.
2. Introduce in the oven at 350 degrees F, bake for 40 minutes, cool down and serve.

Cinnamon Avocado and Berries Mix

Preparation time: 5 minutes

Cooking time: 0 minutes

Servings: 4

Nutritional Values (Per Serving):

- Calories 16
- Fat 8
- Fiber 4.2
- Carbs 12.3
- Protein 8.4

Ingredients:

- 1 cup blackberries
- 1 cup strawberries, halved
- 1 cup avocado, peeled, pitted and cubed

- 1 cup coconut cream
- 1 teaspoon cinnamon powder
- 4 tablespoons stevia

Directions:

1. In a bowl, combine the berries with the avocado and the other ingredients, toss, divide into smaller bowls and serve cold.

Raisins and Berries Cream

Preparation time: 5 minutes

Cooking time: 0

Servings: 4

Nutritional Values (Per Serving):

- Calories 192
- Fat 6.5
- Fiber 3.4
- Carbs 9.5
- Protein 5

Ingredients:

- 1 cup coconut cream
- 1 cup blackberries
- 3 tablespoons stevia
- 2 tablespoons raisins
- 2 tablespoons lime juice

Directions:

1. In a blender, the cream with the berries and the other ingredients except the raisins, pulse well, divide into cups, sprinkle the raisins on top and cool down before serving.

Baked Rhubarb

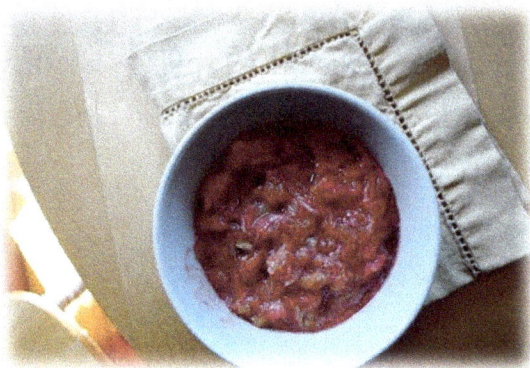

Preparation time: 10 minutes

Cooking time: 20 minutes

Servings: 4

Nutritional Values (Per Serving):

- Calories 176
- Fat 4.5
- Fiber 7.6
- Carbs 11.5
- Protein 5

Ingredients:

- 4 teaspoons stevia
- 1 pound rhubarb, roughly sliced
- 1 teaspoon vanilla extract
- 2 tablespoons avocado oil
- 1 teaspoon cinnamon powder
- 1 teaspoon nutmeg, ground

Directions:

1. Arrange the rhubarb on a baking sheet lined with parchment paper, add the stevia, vanilla and the other ingredienyts, toss and bake at 350 degrees F for 20 minutes.
2. Divide the baked rhubarb into bowls and serve cold.

Curry with Bok Choy

Preparation time: 15 minutes

Cooking time: 15 minutes

Servings: 3

Nutritions:

- Calories: 200
- Total Fats: 15.3g
- Carbohydrates: 13.4g
- Fiber: 4.8g
- Protein: 4.7g
- Sugar: 5.2

Ingredients:

- 2 tablespoons extra virgin coconut oil or olive oil
- 1 small onion, peeled, finely diced

- 2 cloves garlic, peeled, finely chopped
- 1 tablespoon curry powder
- 1 tablespoon fresh grated ginger
- ½ teaspoon ground turmeric
- ½ teaspoon ground fenugreek
- 2 bok choy, washed, feet removed, roughly chopped (14 oz.)
- 14 oz. unsweetened coconut milk
- ½ cup vegetable stock

For serving:

- Lemon juice
- Fresh coriander
- Chili flake

Directions:

1. Place a large skillet over medium heat and add oil. Once the oil is heated, add onions and garlic and cook 1-2 minutes or until golden brown, taking care not to burn them.
2. Add curry powder, grated ginger, turmeric and fenugreek. Stir fry 30 seconds to1 minute until fragrant.

3. Stir in bok choy then cover, turn the heat down to medium-low, and cook 3-4 minutes.
4. Increase the heat to medium-high, uncover and cook 3 - 4 minutes to evaporate the vegetable juice slightly.
5. Pour in coconut milk and vegetable stock; cook an additional 10 minutes until a thick liquid reduces.
6. Place curry in a serving bowl. Drizzle with lemon juice. Sprinkle with freshly chopped coriander and chili flakes.

Zucchini bread

Preparation time: 20 minutes

Cooking time: 50 minutes

Servings: 12

Nutritions:

- Calories: 143
- Total Fats: 13g
- Carbohydrates: 2g
- Fiber: 1g
- Protein: 2g

Ingredients:

For the Loaf:

- 2 cups almond flour
- 2 teaspoons baking powder
- ½ teaspoon xanthan gum
- ¼ teaspoon salt

- ½ cup coconut oil, melted
- ¾ cup Swerve granular
- 3 large eggs
- 1 teaspoon vanilla extract
- 2 tablespoons fresh lemon juice
- 1 tablespoon lemon zest
- 1 cup zucchini shredded, drained

For the Glaze:

- ⅓ cup Swerve confectioners
- 4 tablespoons lemon juice

Directions:

1. Preheat oven to 325°F. Cover the loaf pan with parchment paper.
2. Combine flour, salt, baking powder, and xanthan gum in a bowl. Mix well.
3. In a separate medium bowl, whisk together oil, Swerve granular, eggs, vanilla, and lemon juice.
4. Add the wet **Ingredients:** to the dry **Ingredients:** and mix until just combined.
5. Fold the zucchini and lemon zest into the batter.

6. Pour the batter into the prepared loaf pan and bake until a toothpick inserted into the middle comes out clean, about 50 minutes. If you find your zucchini bread is browning too quickly, you can cover the pan with foil.

7. Remove from the oven and let the bread cool in the pan for 10 minutes. Carefully remove the bread from the pan and cool completely on a wire rack.

8. Whisk together Swerve confectioners and lemon juice. Drizzle loaf with glaze.

9. Slice and serve.

Flax Egg (vegan)

Preparation time: 12 minutes

Cooking time: 0 minute

Servings: 1

Nutritions:

- Calories: 37kcal
- Net Carbs: 0.2g
- Fat: 2.7g
- Protein: 1.1g
- Fiber: 1.9g
- Sugar: 0g

Ingredients:

- 1 tbsp. ground flaxseed
- 2-3 tbsp. lukewarm water

Directions:

1. Mix the ground flaxseed and water in a small bowl by using a spoon.
2. Cover the mixture and let it sit for 10 minutes.
3. Use the flax egg immediately, or, store it in an airtight container in the fridge and consume within 5 days.

Simple Marinara Sauce (vegan)

Preparation time: 10 minutes

Cooking time: 10 minutes

Servings: 8

Nutritions:

- Calories: 23kcal
- Net Carbs: 2.8g
- Fat: 1.1g
- Protein: 0.7g
- Fiber: 0.9g
- Sugar: 0.1g

Ingredients:

- 3 tbsp. olive oil
- 1 14-oz. can peeled tomatoes (no sugar added)
- ⅓ cup red onion (diced)
- 2 garlic cloves (minced)

- 2 tbsp. oregano (fresh and chopped, or 1 tbsp. dried)
- ½ tsp. cayenne pepper
- Optional: 1 tbsp. sunflower seed butter (use grass-fed butter for a lacto sauce)

Directions:

1. Heat the olive oil in a medium-sized skillet over medium heat.
2. Add the onions, garlic, salt, and cayenne pepper. Sauté the onions until translucent while stirring the ingredients.
3. Add the peeled tomatoes and more salt and pepper to taste.
4. Stir the ingredients, cover the skillet, and allow the sauce to softly cook for 10 minutes.
5. Add the oregano, and if desired, stir in the optional butter.
6. Take the skillet off the heat. The sauce is now ready to be used in a recipe!
7. Alternatively, store the sauce in an airtight container in the fridge and consume within 3 days. Store for a maximum of 30 days in the freezer and thaw at room temperature.

Greek Chia Pudding (lacto)

Preparation time: 20 minutes

Cooking time: 0 minute

Servings: 3

Nutritions:

- Calories: 318kcal
- Net Carbs: 6.5g
- Fat: 26.6g
- Protein: 11.9g
- Fiber: 7.4g
- Sugar: 4g

Ingredients:

- 1 cup full-fat Greek yogurt
- ½ cup full-fat coconut milk
- ½ scoop organic soy protein powder (vanilla or chocolate flavor)

- 5 tbsp. chia seeds
- 4-6 drops stevia sweetener (or alternatively, use low-carb maple syrup)
- ¼ cup raspberries
- ¼ cup pecans (crushed)
- Optional: 1-2 tbsp. water

Directions:

1. In a medium-sized bowl, mix the yogurt with the coconut milk.
2. Stir in the protein powder and chia seeds until the protein powder is fully incorporated. Add some water if necessary.
3. Allow the pudding to sit for 2 minutes; then add the stevia sweetener and give the yogurt another stir.
4. Refrigerate the pudding overnight (or for at least 8 hours). This will guarantee a perfect pudding.
5. Top the pudding with the raspberries and crushed pecans; serve and enjoy!
6. Alternatively, store the pudding in an airtight container and keep it in the fridge and consume within 4 days. Or, you can freeze the pudding for a maximum of 30 days and thaw at room temperature.